Real Fo

Infants & Toddlers

let's start out right

Written in collaboration with a board-certified nutritionist, a pediatric cardiologist and an Italian Nonna

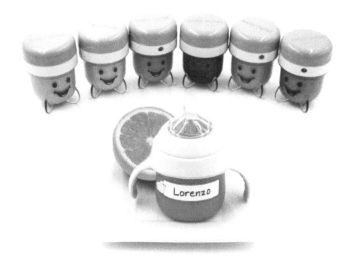

Lorenzo

By Carol Amendola-D'Anca MS, CNS, LDN
With contributions from Barbara J. Deal MD, MS and Raffaella Florio

Real Food for Infants & Toddlers
Carol Amendola-D'Anca
info@foodnotmeds.com

Book Cover Credit: Point9 - Taral Patel
Photo Credit: Giovanni D'Anca

Paperback ISBN: 978-0-578-69021-6

eBook ISBN: 978-0-578-69022-3

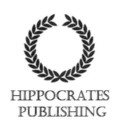

HIPPOCRATES
PUBLISHING

Table of Contents

For the Newest Generation and All Who Nourish Them

Chapter 1:
Culture, Nutrition, and the Standard American Diet

There was a time, not too long ago, when the food we ate did not come in a package. Labels were non-existent, as were the complex ingredient lists we have become accustomed to today. We simply cooked and ate real food.

Infants and children were fed with natural intuition and in the customs of food cultures passed down over hundreds of thousands of years of human evolution and resourcefulness. Food was grown, picked, prepared and eaten without much of the worry over nutrition that we experience today.

Although it's true that life expectancy has risen over the centuries, due to the discovery of antibiotics and the contributions of public health measures, we have now replaced infectious disease with non-communicable diseases including obesity, cardiovascular disease, diabetes and high blood pressure – all affecting children as well as adults today.

While the topic of nutrition and eating well is confusing and hotly debated, there are a few main reasons why our dietary intake has changed dramatically over the past 100 years. Let's briefly explore them to provide a background for feeding our kids well and saving them from the devastation of chronic illnesses that plague our nation today.

Today, diverse food cultures are disappearing at a rapid rate and along with it the cultural knowledge of what to eat, how to grow and prepare food. The speed at which this is happening can destroy the evolution of a food heritage that took place over thousands of years in a couple of generations. When this happens, populations are left with nothing more than heavily processed and manufactured food to try and nourish themselves with food that their ancestors wouldn't even recognize. What we do know is that when people shift away from their traditional diets and toward the Standard American Diet, their health suffers.

This is especially true in the United States, known as the "melting pot" of nations. Immigrants that once followed the diet of their ancestors are quickly assimilating into America's food culture. While it once took at least 2 or 3 generations for food cultures to disappear, today a heritage diet can disappear in as little as a couple of decades.

I offer up my own story leading to my interest in nutrition that is closely related to my cultural heritage. The early years of my life were spent growing up in a heavily populated Italian immigrant community in a small town of about 50,000 people. The section of town I grew up was known as "Little Italy." People that settled in "Little Italy" were recent immigrants. They re-created the only life they knew in the small rural areas of their homeland.

The home I grew up in during my early years was not surrounded by grass. Instead there was a huge garden around every space around our home that my grandfather tended as beautifully as any master gardener today. I grew up very aware of the changing seasons and availability of food throughout the year. We didn't eat fresh strawberries in the winter because they weren't available. Instead we enjoyed beautiful grape jams that were canned when the grapes from our local grapevine ripened. Fall was an especially busy time around my home as I watched my mother and her six sisters cook and preserve foods that we would enjoy throughout the winter.

My middle school years were spent at the local junior high school a few miles from home. I found myself in my own type of cultural melting pot. As I left the safe cultural surroundings of my neighborhood, I began noticing the vast differences between my mother's hand packed Mediterranean lunch and the lunches of white bread sandwiches, sodas and store bought cookies and cakes in the lunches of students all around me. I found it amusing that they could not even identify the foods in my lunch as I opened it each day, mostly dried fruit and apricots, walnuts, maybe a fresh apple, a homemade oatmeal and banana cookie, and water to drink. These very moments of discovery sparked my interest in nutrition and passion for learning and research that continues to this day.

Although some changes are inevitable, fortunately, my family didn't abandon the foods of our culture. There was no need to worry about reading labels, about what to eat, or about what restaurant we were going for dinner. Some of my fondest childhood memories are of spending time in the beautiful garden that nourished not only our bodies but was a way of life rarely duplicated once becoming assimilated to the American way of life.

Lifestyles have changed. While beautiful fruit and vegetable gardens may not surround our homes today, we can still build a healthful food culture for ourselves and for our children. Most importantly we can help our children develop the taste of real food early on in life. Unfortunately, this development can only happen very early in life before a child is exposed to sugary, processed and artificially flavored foods. New mothers, fathers, friends and families have a very short window of opportunity to avoid the addictive onslaught of sugary, artificially flavored, colored and overly processed food.

A wonderful way to begin introducing the tastes, flavor and nutrition in vegetables to infants and toddlers is through creamed vegetables in small amounts. One of the best gifts that moms, families and caregivers can give to infants and toddlers is to assist in introducing the delicious flavors and textures of highly nutritious foods. The recipes in this book from the Italian nonna are the direct result from a cuisine that is most popular, most copied in the world and dating back to the 4th century BC. Yet, as you read through them you will quickly see they are easy to prepare and transport with the baby throughout the day.

Today, depending on which article or study you read, the typical standard American diet is comprised of 50 – 89% of packaged, processed and now a new category, highly processed food. Processing of food removes the fiber, water and most nutrients, those very nutrients required to build a lifetime foundation of health in the lives of infants and toddlers.

The connection between dietary changes and the epidemic of chronic illness including heart disease, diabetes, high blood pressure and some cancers is highly correlated. Increasingly, chronic illness is affecting our children at an earlier age than ever before. Heart disease, diabetes and a myriad of illnesses begin long before they are diagnosed, even beginning in the womb.

Most of us have heard this message, but at the same time, we are faced with the reality that processed food isn't going away anytime soon. It's become embedded in the culture, lifestyle and kitchens of populations living in almost all economically developed countries today. Food and beverage companies have marketing budgets directed specifically at toddlers alone is a whopping $77 million each year! That's $210,000 spent each and every day aimed at marketing unhealthful food to our children. Imagine being a toddler seeing their favorite TV character on a brightly colored box of snacks, cereals and sweets from their seat in a grocery cart and wanting it – all before he or she can even read!

If we are to address this offensive upon the health of our nation, it begins with changes we are willing to make, and it begins with building a strong framework of how our children eat. And, if we are going to affect a change, it's important to start early in a child's life as children become settled in taste preferences by the age of 2 years. Waiting until after they have had their first "smash cake" may already be too late.

You will enjoy reading the chapter by Dr. Barbara Deal, pediatric cardiologist, regarding her findings. You may be surprised to learn that good nutrition for babies, infants and even adults, doesn't begin at birth, but instead while developing in the mother's womb. Some studies suggest tastes start before our babies leave the womb as babies whose mothers ate certain foods during pregnancy or while breastfeeding tended to like these same maternal dietary foods later on. The flavor of foods is reflected in amniotic fluid and in breast milk. What a great opportunity to build a healthy foundation for the baby well before it is born.

References

Nutrients. 2019 Jul 24;11(8). pii: E1704. doi: 10.3390/nu11081704.

The Healthfulness of the US Packaged Food and Beverage Supply: A Cross-Sectional Study.

Baldridge AS[1], Huffman MD[2,3], Taylor F[3], Xavier D[4], Bright B[4], Van Horn LV[2], Neal B[3], Dunford E[3].

Health News, November 1, 2016: Big Money Spent on Marketing Unhealthy baby, toddler foods.

Prenatal and Postnatal Flavor Learning by Human Infants

Julie A. Mennella, Coren P. Jagnow and Gary K. Beauchamp

Pediatrics June 2001, 107 (6) e88; DOI: https://doi.org/10.1542/peds.107.6.e88

Chapter 2:
Raising our children to become the healthiest adults possible

Historically, pediatrics has focused on the care of children with congenital malformations, hereditary diseases, failure to thrive associated with under-nutrition, and infectious diseases. Improved sanitation, antibiotics and immunizations have raised the expectation that almost all children will survive to adulthood.

Now a new type of disease has become prevalent: non-communicable diseases, a cumbersome term for the diseases we acquire due to nutrition and lifestyle: cardiovascular disease including coronary disease, hypertension and stroke, type 2 diabetes, chronic lower respiratory disease, and cancer. In fact, the leading causes of death in the US in 2017 were heart disease, cancer, diabetes, lung disease and stroke. The root cause of non-communicable diseases is an unhealthy diet leading to obesity and contributing to 4 of the top 5 causes of death.(1) Thus, one of the most important ways to raise a child to become a healthy adult is to help children maintain a healthy weight during childhood.

There is a powerful tool to reduce these diseases that does not involve medication or surgery or specialized doctor visits. This tool is healthy nutrition beginning at birth, and once established in early childhood, is a habit of a lifetime. If your child enters kindergarten at a healthy weight, odds are in their favor that they will reach adolescence and adulthood at a healthy weight. (2) For the first 5 to 10 years of life, nutrition is almost completely controlled by parents and family.

Providing your child with healthy nutrition in early childhood is in your hands, and sets the framework for a healthy heart and lifestyle at all ages.

Considering that babies are in general not born overweight, obesity is acquired, often beginning in earliest infancy. Almost 14% of infants and toddlers in the US are obese, increasing to 18% of children 2 -11 years of age, and 21% of adolescents. (3) Presently 40% of adults are obese. (4)Infants who gain weight rapidly, crossing weight percentiles on their growth chart or achieving a weight-for-height ratio >85 percentile, are 2.5 times more likely to have severe obesity by age 6 years. (5)Almost 90% of children who are obese at 3 years of age are obese as adolescents.(6) Among adolescents with obesity, 80% will have obesity in adulthood. Based on current levels of childhood obesity, simulated growth trajectories predict that 57% of today's children will be obese at the age of 35 years. (2) Altering the development of early childhood obesity is thus a major public health policy imperative affecting all areas of adult well-being and life-expectancy.

Rather than a personal cosmetic problem, obesity is a chronic disease that affects all parts of the body and shortens life expectancy, as summarized in **Figure 1.** (7)The stigmatization of obesity begins in early childhood with social isolation, discrimination, and bullying, with subsequent decreased sports participation, orthopedic problems, and depression by early adolescence. (8) Children with obesity have reduced overall academic achievement evident in elementary school years, with deficits in executive functioning, visuo-spatial skills and motor skills. (9) The association of adiposity with childhood and adult asthma is becoming more apparent, worsening asthma attacks and their frequency. (10) Effects of fat tissue on metabolic markers in the blood begins in childhood, with abnormal cholesterol and triglyceride levels, elevated blood pressure, and fatty infiltration of the liver.(11)

Type 2 diabetes, with elevated fasting blood glucose and resistance to the body's insulin, was once a disease diagnosed only in adults. Now type 2 diabetes is detected in almost 5% of adolescents, as early as age 10-14 years.(12) More than 90% of children with type 2 diabetes are obese. These young children's bodies will suffer the effects of abnormal insulin metabolism for many years by the time they reach adulthood, resulting in early onset heart disease. The effects of obesity on the heart and circulation are extensive, including thickening of the heart, premature coronary artery disease, and increased risk for stroke, developing at a much younger age than in previous generations. The age at adverse cardiovascular events, including sudden cardiac death, myocardial infarction, and stroke is decreasing.

The cause of this dramatic increase in obesity is often attributed to larger portion sizes, consumption of highly processed foods, and decreased physical activity. However, the development of obesity in early childhood is more complex, and begins before birth, in utero.(13) Mothers who begin pregnancy obese, with a BMI kg: > 30 kg/m^2, are at increased risk for babies who will become obese children, and obese adults. (14)Maternal obesity causes metabolic and genetic changes in the fetus, causing an increased number of fat cells and propensity to become obese, which may then be transmitted to subsequent generations. Thus, entering pregnancy at an ideal body weight is one of the most important measures to ensure a healthy body weight for the future baby. During pregnancy, maternal smoking, gestational diabetes, and an unhealthy diet can contribute to obesity in offspring. The risks associated with alcohol consumption during pregnancy have been widely publicized. However, there is recent evidence from the Canadian Healthy Infant Longitudinal Development Study that the daily consumption of sugar-sweetened beverages *during pregnancy* is associated with a 2-fold increase in risk for overweight infants at one year of age, and in another study is associated with obesity at age 7 years. (15, 16)

Infants born weighing more than 4 kg (8 pounds 8 oz.), and more importantly, infants with rapid weight gain in the first year of life are at increased risk for development of childhood obesity. After birth, multiple exposures to broad spectrum antibiotics during the first year of life is associated with obesity in some but not all studies.(17) Breastfeeding for the first 4-6 months of life is associated with reduced risk of obesity in childhood.(18) Among other differences, infant formula has a higher protein content than breastmilk, which is believed to contribute to more rapid weight gain in infancy. Each additional week that an infant breastfeeds adds to the protective effect of breastmilk on childhood obesity.

Optimizing nutrition in the first years of life is essential for healthy growth and avoiding early childhood obesity. (19) Sugar-sweetened beverage consumption and added sugars in baked goods contribute significantly to the causes of overweight in children and adults.(20, 21) **Sugar-sweetened beverages** such as soda have no nutritional value, yet they are consumed daily by over 40% of children under the age of 2 years. More than half—60%-of added sugars in the diet of children come from beverages, accounting for almost 19% of total calories for 2-18-year-old youth. (22)In an analysis of dietary contributions to heart disease, sugar-sweetened beverages and processed meats were the 2 most important dietary culprits in adults under age 44 years developing heart disease. (23) **Fruit juices** for children contribute sugars without dietary fiber, which slows the absorption of the sugar; it is recommended that juice intake be limited to < 4-6 ounces daily for children under 6 years, and < 8-12 ounces of daily for older children. (24) See **Table 1** for selected nutritional targets.

Figure 1: Childhood obesity is a disease of a lifetime (7, 8)

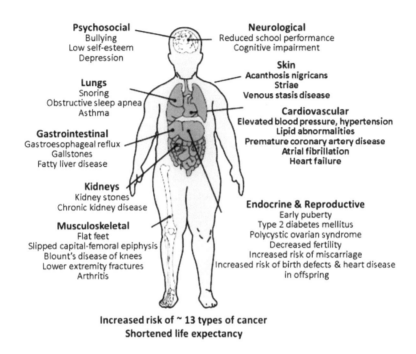

Psychosocial
Bullying
Low self-esteem
Depression

Neurological
Reduced school performance
Cognitive impairment

Skin
Acanthosis nigricans
Striae
Venous stasis disease

Lungs
Snoring
Obstructive sleep apnea
Asthma

Cardiovascular
Elevated blood pressure, hypertension
Lipid abnormalities
Premature coronary artery disease
Atrial fibrillation
Heart failure

Gastrointestinal
Gastroesophageal reflux
Gallstones
Fatty liver disease

Kidneys
Kidney stones
Chronic kidney disease

Endocrine & Reproductive
Early puberty
Type 2 diabetes mellitus
Polycystic ovarian syndrome
Decreased fertility
Increased risk of miscarriage
Increased risk of birth defects & heart disease
in offspring

Musculoskeletal
Flat feet
Slipped capital-femoral epiphysis
Blount's disease of knees
Lower extremity fractures
Arthritis

Increased risk of ~ 13 types of cancer
Shortened life expectancy

Figure modified from Ebbeling CB, et al, Lancet. 2002;360(9331):473-82.

Other foods to limit or avoid include **processed meats** and **ultra-processed foods.** Processed meats include hot dogs, sausages, bacon and ham; these are classified as having cancer-causing potential by the World Health Organization. Additionally, after sugar-

15

sweetened beverages, processed meats are a major contributor to cardiovascular disease in young adults. Ultra-processed foods are defined as "ready to eat" and microwaveable foods, such as breakfast cereals, instant noodles, chicken or fish nuggets, chips, candies, and artificially sweetened beverages. Ultra-processed foods are high in calories, and are made tasty by the addition of sugars, salt, saturated and trans fats; they are easy to consume, low-cost, and low in nutrients, and contribute to both weight gain and cardiovascular disease. Ultra-processed foods are estimated to contribute almost 50% of daily caloric intake, and advertising for these 'food-like substances' specifically target youth. Exchanging consumption of ultra-processed foods for fruits and vegetables can be expected to reduce obesity, type 2 diabetes, and cardiovascular disease. (25, 26)

Healthy eating does not have to be complicated, and does not require a lot of studying. Healthy eating does require being conscious of what you and your child are eating, every day. Focus on the big picture of eating fresh whole foods daily and avoiding highly processed foods and sugar-sweetened beverages. Spend your extra time enjoying each other and physical activity, especially outdoors! Making an effort to share breakfasts and dinner time on a regular basis is an important component of health eating habits. As working parents with children in competitive sports practices, we made the effort to shift dinner-time later in the day, so that my husband and I could sit together with our daughters for at least 15-20 minutes daily.

Guidelines for establishing healthful nutrition for children

Start early! In fact, begin before your baby is born, if possible. **Entering pregnancy at an ideal body mass index** is one of the most significant ways to ensure the best start in life for your offspring. **Breastfeeding exclusively** for the first 4-6 months of life is associated with healthy body weight later in life, not to mention reducing the risk of infection for the baby. Breastfeeding provides optimal nutrition for the growing infant.

Offer/drink water or milk daily. The important message here is to avoid the habit of drinking packaged juices, which provide calories and rapid sugar intake, and develop a taste for sweetness. The American Academy of Pediatrics recommends that young infants under one year of age consume breast milk or infant formula, and avoid cow's milk in the first year of life. Flavored milks contain significant amounts of added sugars and are not recommended. Juice is not recommended under 6 months of age, and should not exceed 4-6 ounces daily for the first 6 years of life, and limiting to under 8-12 ounces daily for older children. Sports drinks are high in added sugars, and are not recommended over water, with the exception of situations where electrolyte repletion is needed; in these situations, dilution to half-strength or less is suitable.

Offer/eat fresh whole foods. Ask the question, would my grandmother recognize this item as food? Fresh whole foods are those grown in the ground, not those manufactured and packaged with a bar code label. When eating packaged foods, check the label: ideally there are fewer than 3-5 ingredients. More than a few ingredients usually means additives or "food-like substitutes" are inside.

Offer/eat at least one serving of fresh fruit every day. Beginning of life-long habit of eating fruits every day at a young age is important. Remember that whole fruits provide necessary fiber, which slows sugar absorption, increases satiety, and lowers blood cholesterol. Fruit juices usually do not have the same fiber content as the fruit, and the sugars are absorbed more rapidly into the bloodstream, eliciting an insulin response from the pancreas, similar to sugar-sweetened beverages.

Offer/eat vegetables daily. Frozen vegetables and fruits retain the nutritional value of fresh produce and offer convenience and longer "shelf-life". Microwaving vegetables is also good for retaining nutritional value. "Eat the rainbow" is the reminder to choose brightly colored vegetables for added nutritional value: dark-green, red, orange, yellow.

Offer/consume whole grains daily. In general, avoiding white foods works for grains: 100% whole grain rather than white bread; brown rather than white rice, sweet rather than white potatoes. Look for "100% whole grain/wheat" on the label, rather than labels that state "contains whole grains". Boxed cereals can be a major source of added sugars, which are marketed to young children. Terms such as "honey", "frosted", "golden" are tip-offs to high sugar content. Read cereal labels, and choose cereals with less than 6-8 grams of sugar/serving, and containing at least 3 grams of fiber/serving. Oatmeal with added fresh fruit is a good choice! For older children and adolescents, popcorn is a good source of fiber without added fats; caution is needed to avoid popcorn around small children, due to the risk of choking.

Limit consumption of processed meats. Processed meats include hot dogs, sausage, bacon, ham, bologna and other deli-meats. These meats are associated with the development of cardiovascular disease, and are linked to the development of colon cancer. Enough said.

Limit added sugars in the diet. Added sugars in the diet are thought to be the major contributor to the development of metabolic and cardiovascular disease around the world. Added sugars are those not found naturally in food, but are added during preparation. The World Health Organization suggests limiting sugar to less than 5% of total caloric intake for children, which translates into **less than 3**

teaspoons, or less than 12 grams of added sugars daily.(27) Adult women should consume less than 25 grams of added sugars, and adult males, less than 37.5 grams daily according the American Heart Association.(28) For reference, a 12-ounce serving of soda contains approximately 39 grams of sugar. Sugar is sugar regardless of its name: sugar, fructose, brown sugar, agave, honey, maple syrup, coconut sugar, raw sugar, etc.

For adolescents and adults, increased consumption of nuts and seeds (less than one-ounce servings) on a daily basis is healthy. Contrary to public opinion, daily consumption of nuts and seeds is associated with a healthy weight, not weight gain. Of course, nuts can pose a choking risk for young children, and should be avoided in this age group and in the setting of allergies. Nuts and seeds are rich in mono- and poly-unsaturated fats, which are healthy and recommended as part of a heart-healthy diet.(29)

The first 1000 days of life are considered crucial to developing a lifetime of health by optimizing nutrition.(30) Every effort you can make to establish healthy eating habits during early childhood will pay enormous dividends in giving your child the best opportunity to become the healthiest adult possible. And after all, isn't this is one of our major goals as parents?

OPTIMAL TARGETS FOR HEALTHY NUTRITION

Time period	Target	Comments
Pregnancy	Achieve and maintain a healthy weight prior to pregnancy	A BMI between 18.5 - 25 kg/m^2 is considered ideal
	Healthy eating during pregnancy	Avoid sugar sweetened beverages and cigarettes
Infancy	Breastfeeding for the first 4-6 months of life	Delay introduction of solid foods until 4-6 months of age
Childhood	Eat real 'whole foods'	Foods without a bar-code are healthiest!
	Avoid sugar sweetened beverages	High in added sugars and calories, contribute to obesity
	Eat a piece of fresh fruit daily	Whole fruit is preferred over fruit juices for the fiber content, and reduced sugar absorption
	Avoid processed meats: bacon, sausage, ham, hot dogs	Associated with cardiovascular disease, and cancers
	Consume whole grains and fiber	Target > 14 grams of fiber daily
	Limit added sugars	Target < 12 grams /daily of added sugar for young children (< 3 teaspoons)

Resources for Nutrition

US Department of Health and Human Services. 2015-2020 Dietary guidelines for Americans. Available for free download at http://health.gov/dietaryguidelines/2015/guidelines.

Gidding SS, Dennison BA, Birch LL, et al. Dietary recommendations for children and adolescents: a guide for practitioners. Pediatrics. 2006 Feb 1;117(2):544-59.

Mozaffarian D, Appel LJ, Van Horn L. Components of a cardioprotective diet: new insights. Circulation. 2011 Jun 21;123(24):2870-91.

Van Horn L, Carson JA, Appel LJ,et al. Recommended dietary pattern to achieve adherence to the American Heart Association/American College of Cardiology (AHA/ACC) guidelines: a scientific statement from the American Heart Association. Circulation. 2016 Nov 29;134(22):e505-29.

Pollan M. Food rules: An eater's manual. Penguin Group USA; 2013.

George Mateljan. The World's Healthiest Foods. website: www.whfoods.org

References

1. Afshin A, Micha R, Webb M, Capewell S, Whitsel L, Rubinstein A, et al. Effectiveness of dietary policies to reduce noncommunicable diseases. In: rd, Prabhakaran D, Anand S, Gaziano TA, Mbanya JC, Wu Y, et al., editors. Cardiovascular, respiratory, and related disorders. Washington (DC)2017.

2. Ward ZJ, Long MW, Resch SC, Giles CM, Cradock AL, Gortmaker SL. Simulation of growth trajectories of childhood obesity into adulthood. N Engl J Med. 2017;377(22):2145-53.

3. Skinner AC, Ravanbakht SN, Skelton JA, Perrin EM, Armstrong SC. Prevalence of obesity and severe obesity in US children, 1999-2016. Pediatrics. 2018;141(3):220173459.

4. Hales CM CM, Fryar CD, Ogden CL. . Prevalence of obesity among adults and youth: United States, 2015-2016. . In: Statistics NCfH, editor. Hyattsville, MD: National Center for Health Statistics; 2017.

5. Nader PR, O'Brien M, Houts R, Bradley R, Belsky J, Crosnoe R, et al. Identifying risk for obesity in early childhood. Pediatrics. 2006;118(3):e594-601.

6. Geserick M, Vogel M, Gausche R, Lipek T, Spielau U, Keller E, et al. Acceleration of bmi in early childhood and risk of sustained obesity. N Engl J Med. 2018;379(14):1303-12.

7. Kelsey MM, Zaepfel A, Bjornstad P, Nadeau KJ. Age-related consequences of childhood obesity. Gerontology. 2014;60(3):222-8.

8. Morales DX, Prieto N, Grineski SE, Collins TW. Race/ethnicity, obesity, and the risk of being verbally bullied: A national multilevel study. Journal of racial and ethnic health disparities. 2019;6(2):245-53.

9. Li N, Yolton K, Lanphear BP, Chen A, Kalkwarf HJ, Braun JM. Impact of early-life weight status on cognitive abilities in children. Obesity (Silver Spring). 2018;26(6):1088-95.

10. Azizpour Y, Delpisheh A, Montazeri Z, Sayehmiri K, Darabi B. Effect of childhood bmi on asthma: A systematic review and meta-analysis of case-control studies. BMC Pediatr. 2018;18(1):143.

11. Turer CB, Brady TM, de Ferranti SD. Obesity, hypertension, and dyslipidemia in childhood are key modifiable antecedents of adult cardiovascular disease: A call to action. Circulation. 2018;137(12):1256-9.

12. Mayer-Davis EJ, Lawrence JM, Dabelea D, Divers J, Isom S, Dolan L, et al. Incidence trends of type 1 and type 2 diabetes among youths, 2002-2012. N Engl J Med. 2017;376(15):1419-29.

13. Fleming TP, Watkins AJ, Velazquez MA, Mathers JC, Prentice AM, Stephenson J, et al. Origins of lifetime health around the time of conception: Causes and consequences. Lancet. 2018;391(10132):1842-52.

14. Voerman E, Santos S, Patro Golab B, Amiano P, Ballester F, Barros H, et al. Maternal body mass index, gestational weight gain, and the risk of overweight and obesity across childhood: An individual participant data meta-analysis. PLoS Med. 2019;16(2):e1002744.

15. Azad MB, Sharma AK, de Souza RJ, Dolinsky VW, Becker AB, Mandhane PJ, et al. Association between artificially sweetened beverage consumption during pregnancy and infant body mass index. JAMA Pediatr. 2016;170(7):662-70.

16. Zhu Y, Olsen SF, Mendola P, Halldorsson TI, Rawal S, Hinkle SN, et al. Maternal consumption of artificially sweetened beverages during pregnancy, and offspring growth through 7 years of age: A prospective cohort study. Int J Epidemiol. 2017;46(5):1499-508.

17. Dawson-Hahn EE, Rhee KE. The association between antibiotics in the first year of life and child growth trajectory. BMC Pediatr. 2019;19(1):23.

18. Rito AI, Buoncristiano M, Spinelli A, Salanave B, Kunesova M, Hejgaard T, et al. Association between characteristics at birth, breastfeeding and obesity in 22 countries: The who european childhood obesity surveillance initiative - cosi 2015/2017. Obes Facts. 2019;12(2):226-43.

19. Schwarzenberg SJ, Georgieff MK. Advocacy for improving nutrition in the first 1000 days to support childhood development and adult health. Pediatrics. 2018;141(2).

20. Luger M, Lafontan M, Bes-Rastrollo M, Winzer E, Yumuk V, Farpour-Lambert N. Sugar-sweetened beverages and weight gain in children and adults: A systematic review from 2013 to 2015 and a comparison with previous studies. Obes Facts. 2017;10(6):674-93.

21. Guasch-Ferre M, Hu FB. Are fruit juices just as unhealthy as sugar-sweetened beverages? JAMA network open. 2019;2(5):e193109.

22. U.S. Department of Health and Human Services and U.S. Department of Agriculture. 2015-2020 Dietary Guidelines for Americans, 8th edition. 2015

23. Micha R, Penalvo JL, Cudhea F, Imamura F, Rehm CD, Mozaffarian D. Association between dietary factors and mortality from heart disease, stroke, and type 2 diabetes in the United States. JAMA. 2017;317(9):912-24.

24. Heyman MB, Abrams SA, Section On Gastroenterology H, Nutrition, Committee On N. Fruit juice in infants, children, and adolescents: Current recommendations. Pediatrics. 2017;139(6):1-10.

25. Poti JM, Braga B, Qin B. Ultra-processed food intake and obesity: What really matters for health-processing or nutrient content? Current obesity reports. 2017;6(4):420-31.

26. Taveras EM. Childhood obesity risk and prevention: Shining a lens on the first 1000 days. Childhood obesity (Print). 2016;12(3):159-61.

27. World Health Organization. Guideline: Sugars intake for adults and children. 2015.

28. Vos MB, Kaar JL, Welsh JA, Van Horn LV, Feig DI, Anderson CAM, et al. Added sugars and cardiovascular disease risk in children: A scientific statement from the American heart association. Circulation. 2017;135(19):e1017-e34.

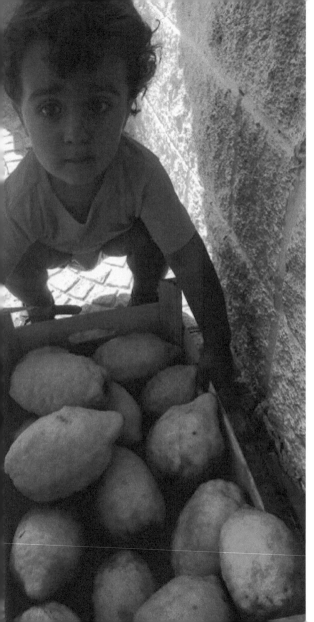

29. Afshin A, Micha R, Khatibzadeh S, Mozaffarian D. Consumption of nuts and legumes and risk of incident ischemic heart disease, stroke, and diabetes: A systematic review and meta-analysis. Am J Clin Nutr. 2014;100(1):278-88.

30. Pietrobelli A, Agosti M. Nutrition in the first 1000 days: Ten practices to minimize obesity emerging from published science. Int J Environ Res Public Health. 2017;14(12).

Chapter 3:

Recipes for Children

6 months to 1 year

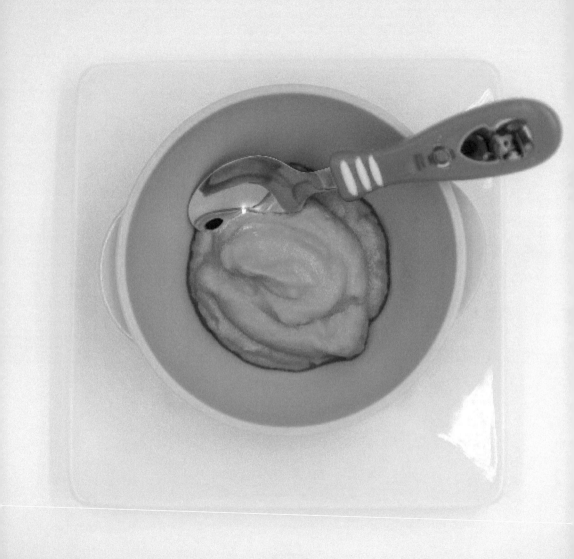

Sweet Potato Pudding

Age to start: 4 – 5 months

Ingredients:

One small sweet potato

Note: you can also use about 1 cup of cubed butternut squash

1/3 c. breast milk

Directions:

If using sweet potato, wash and rub the skin well

If using cubed butternut squash, the outer peel is removed

Place the potato or squash in a baking dish with about 2" of water on the bottom of the dish

Cover the baking dish with foil.

Bake in the oven at 350 degrees for about 30 minutes or until the vegetable is soft when pierced with a fork and feels soft.

When done, remove from the pan and remove the skin of the sweet potato.

Place in blender and process.

Serve as a pudding to the baby

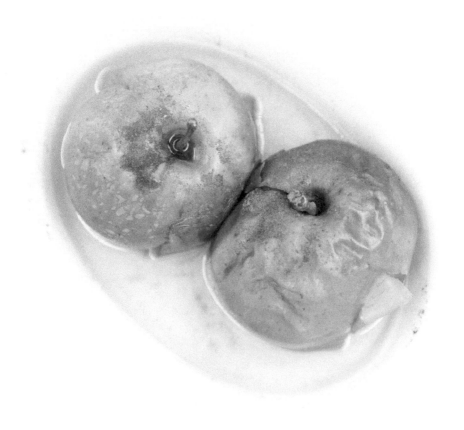

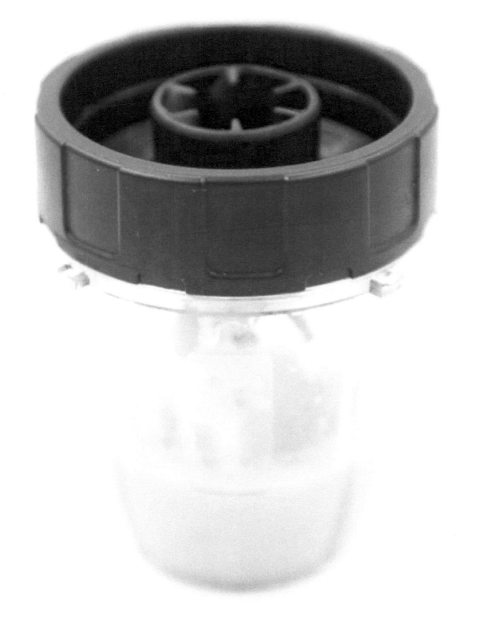

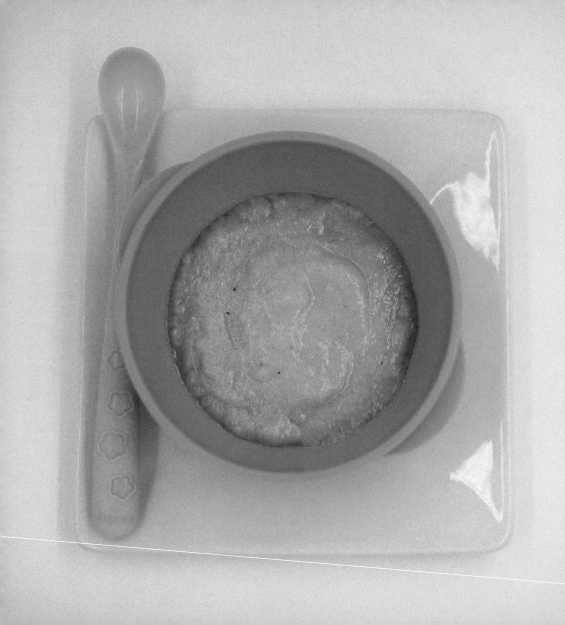

Apple and Cinnamon Puree

When to start feeding; 4-5 months

Ingredients:

1 fully ripe apple – your choice of type. A recommendation is not to use overly tart apples. Mild flavor red apples work well. If the apple is not completely ripe when purchased, place it in a brown paper bag for a couple of days to insure it is ready for eating.

Note: You can substitute a fully ripe pear for the apple for variety.

Cinnamon to sprinkle

Directions:

Place the apple in a baking dish with about 2" of water. Use bottled Acqua Panna Water if available or any good bottled water.

Bake at 350 degrees until the fruit is soft.

Remove the peel and put in the blender.

Place the soft fruit and the water from baking in the blender and blend well.

Sprinkle lightly with cinnamon.

This puree can also be mixed with 1 tablespoon of rice or oatmeal for a morning breakfast.

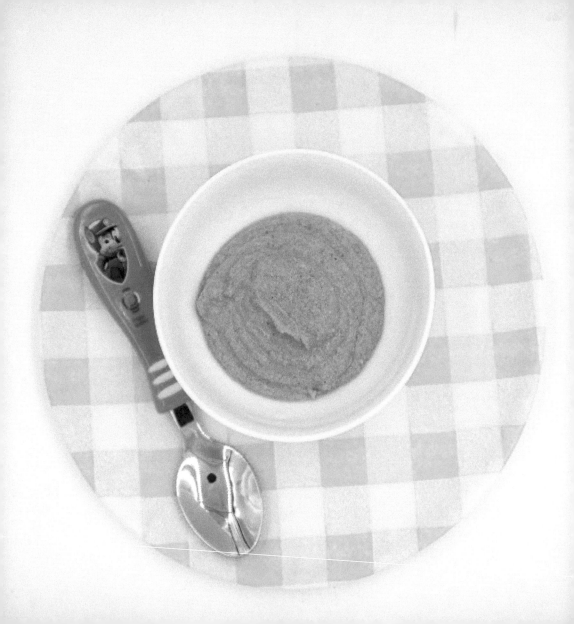

Cream of Peas and Rice

Begin at 6 months

Ingredients:

½ **c** frozen peas (preferably organic)

I t. rice cereal

1/3 c breast milk

1 t. extra virgin olive oil

Directions:

Cover the frozen peas with water in a small saucepan. Cook until soft.

Drain the peas and blend preferable with breast milk or formula if using or water.

Blend together until creamy

Blend together with the rice.

If preferred, season with a very small amount of extra virgin olive oil.

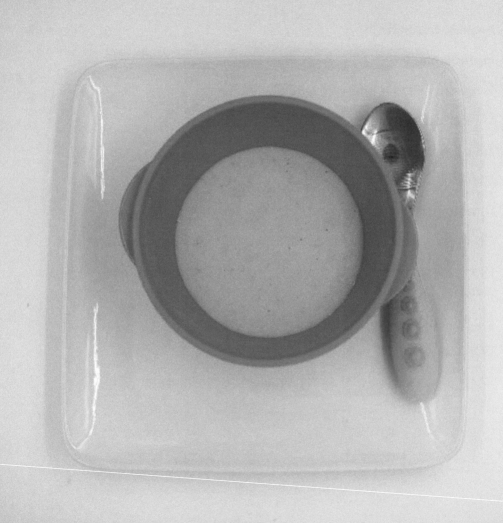

Cream of Corn

Start at 6 months

Ingredients:

1c non gmo corn – fresh or frozen

1/3c mother's breast milk

Directions:

Place the corn in a small saucepan and cover with water.

Cook until tender – about 15 minutes

When the corn is soft, place in the blender with the milk

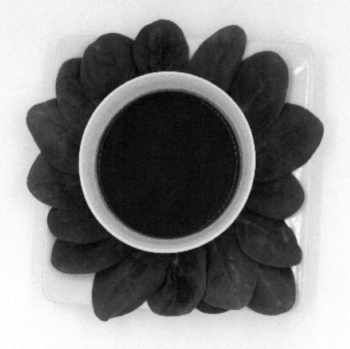

Veggie Lentil Puree

Start at 8 or 9 months

Ingredients:

¼ cup lentils

½ potato

1 small carrot

1 t. extra virgin olive oil

Directions:

Rinse the lentils, carrot and potato well

Peel the potato and cut into ½" pieces

Brush the carrot clean and peel – cut into small pieces

Place the above ingredients in a heavy bottom saucepan and cover with water.

Bring to a boil, then reduce heat and simmer for about 30 minutes or until the water is absorbed and lentils are tender.

Place everything in a food mill or blender and blend well.

Soup is ready to serve the baby.

Yogurt and Apple

Start at 8 months

Ingredients:

One medium-sized golden apple

200 ml of organic apple juice

Half a jar of plain yogurt – organic, read the label to insure it doesn't contain additives.

Directions:

Wash the apple well, dry and peel.

Divide it into quarters, remove the inner core and cut into chunks.

Put the pieces of apple in a saucepan, cover them with the apple juice and cook for about ten minutes or until the pieces of apple flake.

Pour everything into a small bowl, crush with a fork, let cool and add the white yogurt, mixing well.

Serve the baby.

Note: Substitute strawberries, blueberries or other fruits for the apple

Snack

Start at 5-6 months

Ingredients:

½ c. fresh blueberries (or frozen thawed) Organic with either option

1/3 c. water or breast milk

1 t. rice cereal

Blend in blender or immersion blender

Note:

At 12 months you can substitute 1/3 c. plain yogurt in this recipe to make a yogurt snack.

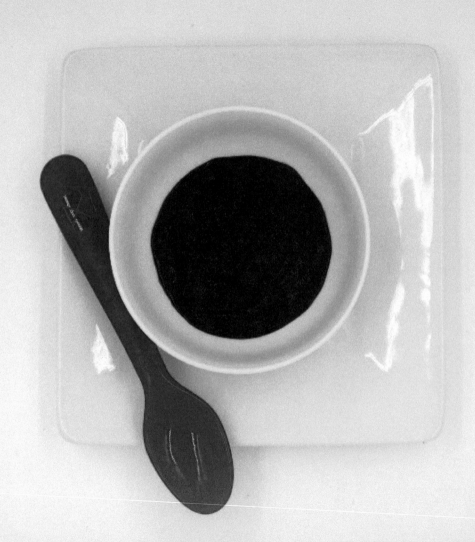

Pureed Beets

Start at 10 months

Ingredients:

2 small beets, washed well, leave skin on

Directions:

Boil the whole beets in a small amount of water for about 20 minutes or until soft when pierced with a fork or knife.

Allow the beets to cool, remove the skin

Place in the blender with small amount of the cooking water or breast milk

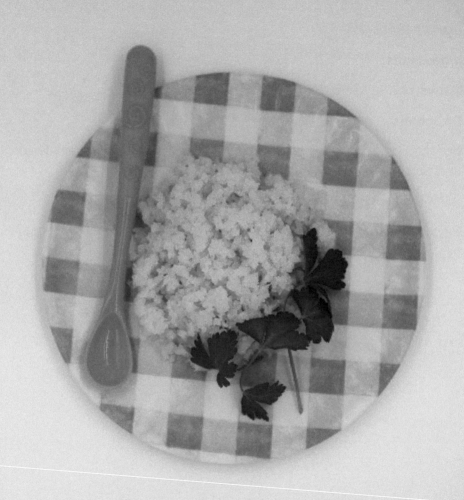

Cream of Cauliflower

Start at 8- to 10-months-old

Wash and cut 1 cup of white cauliflower

Bring to a boil in a pan covered with water for 15 minutes until soft and tender.

Drain and transfer in a food processor or blender until smooth.

Use the cooking water as needed to reach desired consistency; use breast milk or formula in place of water for a creamier texture.

When the baby is ready for finger foods, you can serve whole cauliflower florets cut into tiny pieces.

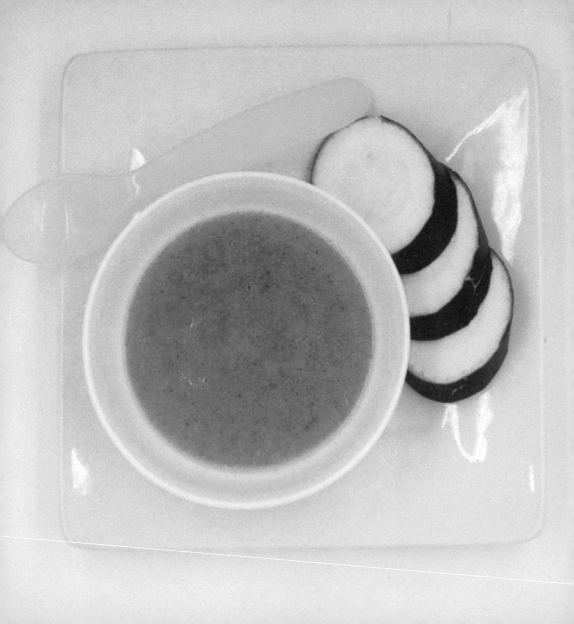

Minestrina

8 or 9 months

Ingredients:

1 small zucchini

½ potato

½ carrot

1 T rice cereal

1 t. extra virgin olive oil

½ liter baby water

Directions:

Wash the zucchini, potato and carrot well.

Cut the vegetables in 1 - 11/2" pieces and place in a heavy bottom pan.

Add the water.

Cook the vegetables for about 30 minutes until tender.

When tender, process the vegetables in a food mill.

Pour into a serving dish. Add some of the cooking water if needed to thin it out.

Mix well. Drizzle the teaspoon of EVOO and serve.

Note:

You can vary the basic recipe above using vegetable broth instead of water

Smoothie of Banana & Apple

We have this one twice

Ingredients:

Small peeled and diced apple

½ small banana cut in pieces

75 gr water a few drops of lemon juice

Directions:

Bring the water in a small saucepan to a boil. Add the lemon, apple and banana and cook for 5 minutes.

At the end of cooking, move it all in a blender and blend well.

Serve as a snack or following a meal

Cream of Vegetables

Start at 9 months

Ingredients:

Zucchini - chopped

Carrots – chopped

Baby spinach

Directions:

Place all vegetables in a small pan and cover with ½ cup of vegetable broth

When vegetables are soft, place in blender

Can make a veggie pop by placing in the freezer. These are great for when teething or for a snack.

Can also make fruit and yogurt pops

Chapter 4:

Recipes for Children

1 year and Beyond

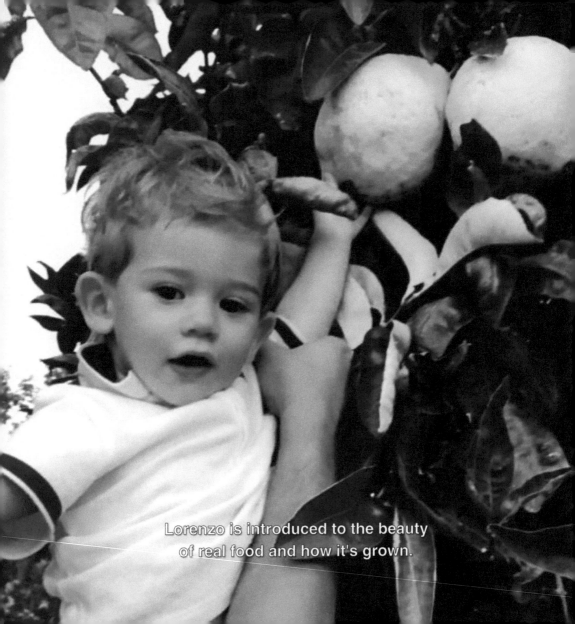

Lorenzo is introduced to the beauty
of real food and how it's grown.

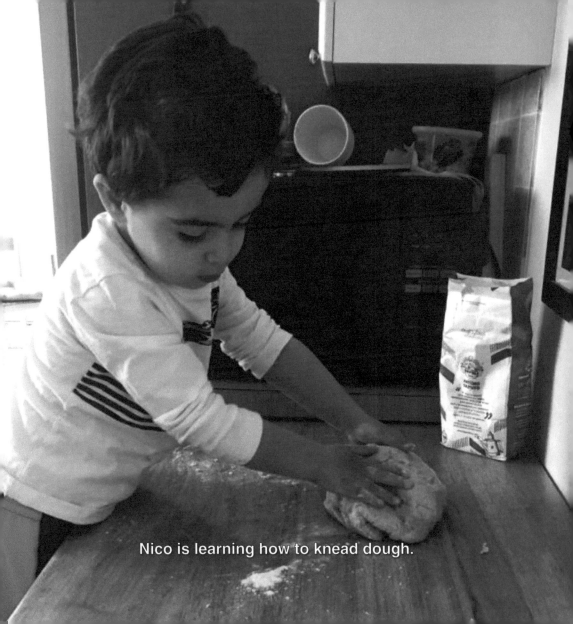
Nico is learning how to knead dough.

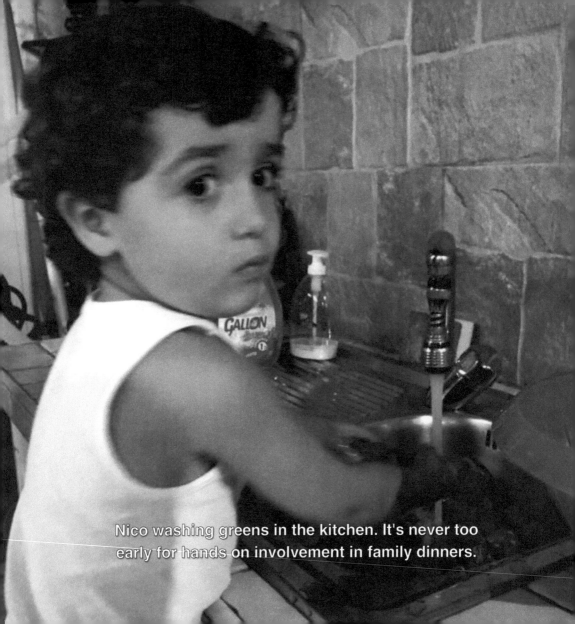

Nico washing greens in the kitchen. It's never too early for hands on involvement in family dinners.

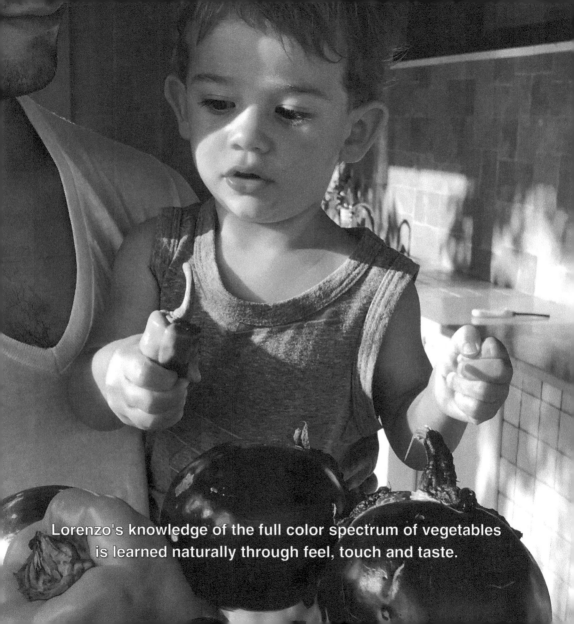

Lorenzo's knowledge of the full color spectrum of vegetables is learned naturally through feel, touch and taste.

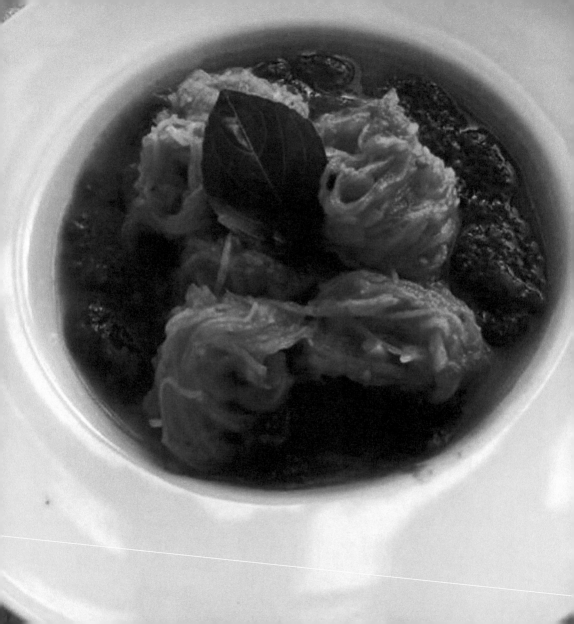

Roasted spaghetti squash with marinara sauce.

1 medium spaghetti squash wash well. Place entire squash in a roster pan in the oven at 350 for 20 minutes.

Take out the oven and let cool off.

Cut the squash in half. Clean out the seeds and with a fork, then scrape across the squash to form spaghetti like strands.

For the sauce:

1 can San Marzano peeled tomatoes

1 scallion

2 tablespoons of Evo extra virgin olive oil

1 teaspoon salt

1/4 cup fresh basil

Heat the olive oil with the chopped scallion add the tomatoes and salt let the sauce cook for 10 minutes. At the end add the fresh chopped basil.

Put the spaghetti squash in a big bowl add the sauce and mix together.

Optional you can sprinkle with parmigiano reggiano cheese.

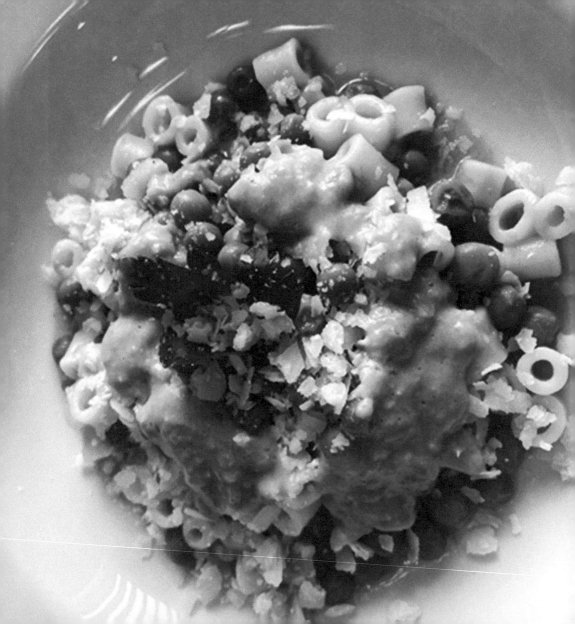

Pasta with Peas

Ingredients:

1 cup of frozen peas

1 scallion finely chopped

2 tablespoons of EVOO

1 teaspoon of finely chopped fresh parsley

Suggested pasta tubettini/ditalini or a small pasta of your choice

Pinch of salt

1 tablespoon of grated parmigiano reggiano cheese

Directions:

1. Bring 6 cups of water to boil for pasta. Once pasta boils add a pinch of salt.

2. While water is boiling, warm up EVOO with scallions in a pan for 2 minutes.

3. Add frozen peas to the pan and cover for 5 minutes. Add a pinch of salt.

4. Add 1/3 cup of boiling water from the pasta pan to the peas for moisture. Cover pan for 5 more minutes.

5. Drain pasta and keep ½ cup of water aside for additional cream, and move pasta to a bowl.

6. Take 2 tablespoons of cooked peas (include water and scallions) and puree in a blender.

7. Mix pasta, peas, and cream of peas together in a bowl (if necessary add additional water to make creamy consistency).

8. Optional: Garnish with grated fresh parmigiano reggiano and fresh parsley.

Veggie sticks

Ingredients:

1 zucchini

1 carrot (pre-boiled)

1 potato

EVOO, as needed

1 cup bread crumbs

1 tbsp grated Parmigiano reggiano

Directions:

Preheat oven to 350 degrees.

Slice the vegetables lengthwise (julienne style) about ¼ inch thick.

Toss vegetable sticks with a drizzle of EVOO, and toss with bread crumbs to coat.

Place vegetable sticks on a cookie sheet lined with parchment paper and cook for 15 minutes.

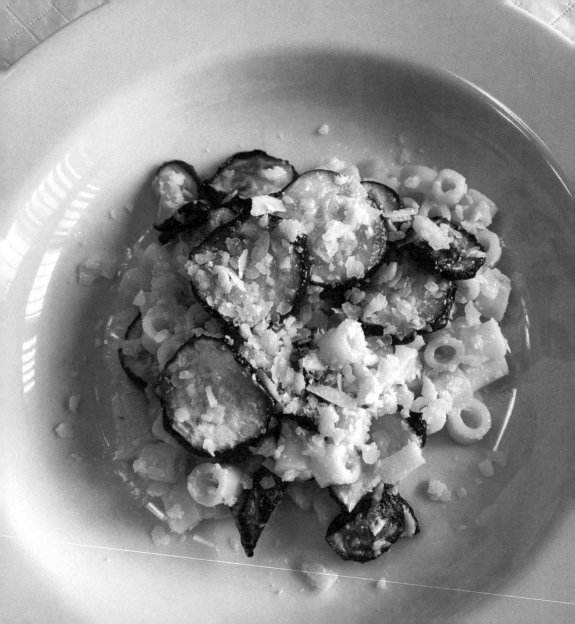

Pasta with Zucchini

Ingredients:

2 (medium) Zucchini, sliced finely

2 tablespoons of EVOO

1 teaspoon of finely chopped fresh parsley

Suggested pasta tubettini/ditalini or a small pasta of your choice

Pinch of salt

1 tablespoon of grated parmigiano reggiano cheese

Directions:

Bring 6 cups of water to boil for pasta. Once pasta boils add a pinch of salt.

While water is boiling, warm up EVOO, then add sliced zucchini to a pan stirring occasionally until golden brown (about 8-10 minutes).

Drain pasta and transfer to a bowl.

Add zucchini to pasta and mix together.

Optional: Garnish with grated fresh parmigiano reggiano and fresh parsley.

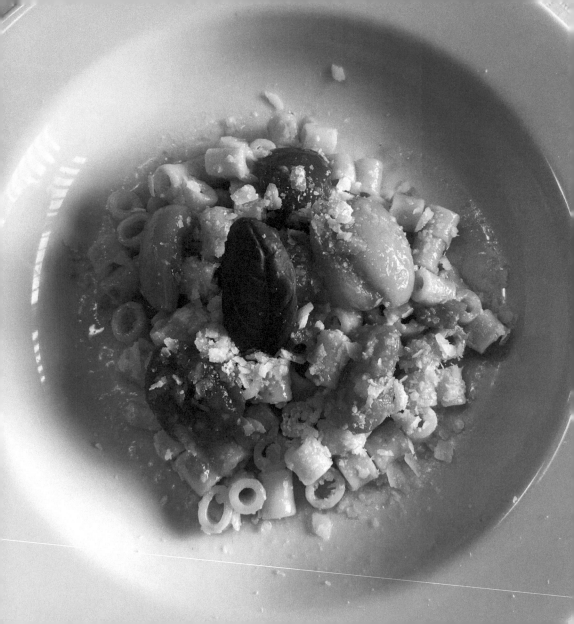

Pasta with Rainbow Cherry Tomato sauce

Ingredients:

2 cups of Rainbow Cherry Tomatoes (cut in half)

3 tablespoons of EVOO

1 clove of garlic, minced

Fresh basil to garnish

Suggested pasta tubettini/ditalini or a small pasta of your choice

Pinch of salt

1 tablespoon of grated parmigiano reggiano cheese

Directions:

Bring 6 cups of water to boil for pasta. Once pasta boils add salt.

While water is boiling, warm up EVOO, then add sliced Rainbow cherry tomatoes to the pan stirring occasionally until tomatoes are tender and a sauce forms (about 10 minutes).

Drain pasta and transfer to a bowl.

Add Rainbow cherry tomato sauce to pasta and mix together.

Optional: Garnish with grated fresh parmigiano reggiano and fresh basil.

Grilled Apple and Pear slices

Ingredients:

Slice 1 apple and 1 pear (½ inch thick)

1 tbsp coconut oil , melted

1 tsp cinnamon

Directions:

Heat grill pan until hot.

Place sliced apple and pear on the grill pan. Turn once grill lines appear to cook on the other side.

Remove slices to a dish and toss with coconut oil and sprinkle with cinnamon.

Serve immediately or refrigerate for a snack.

Cucumber and Blood Orange Salad

Ingredients:

1 English cucumber, sliced finely

1 Blood orange, cut into chunks

1 Tbsp. EVOO

1 tsp. Of White Vinegar glaze

Directions:

Cut English cucumber and Blood orange into age appropriate sizes.

Mix the ingredients together.

Strawberry Frozen Yogurt Popsicles

Ingredients:

1 cup of fresh strawberries

½ cup of plain greek yogurt

½ tsp of lemon juice

Popsicle mold

Directions:

Add all ingredients into the blender. Blend until all strawberries are pureed.

Transfer mixture to popsicle molds (you can be creative and find different shapes for children) or freezer safe cups.

Place it into the freezer for 3-4 hours.

Homemade Pesto

Ingredients:

1 cup of basil leaves, washed and dried

¼ cup of EVOO

1 clove of garlic

¼ cup of pine nuts

Pinch of salt

½ cup of grated parmigiano reggiano cheese

Directions:

Blend basil leaves, EVOO, garlic and pine nuts in a food processor until a smooth texture is obtained.

Transfer to a mixing bowl, add salt and cheese to the mixture. If needed extra EVOO may be added for a smoother consistency,

Sauce may be stored in small jars. Top with EVOO to cover and keep pesto up to a month in the refrigerator.

Pesto may be added to various dishes, such as pasta, quinoa, bruschetta, chicken, tomatoes, etc.

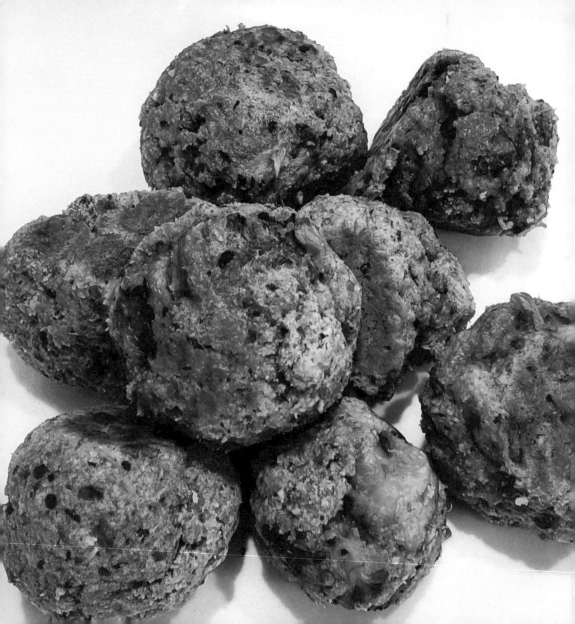

Eggplant balls

Ingredients:

2 medium eggplant

EVOO

1 cup of bread crumbs

2 eggs

½ cup of parmigiano reggiano (or pecorino romano cheese) , grated

1 tablespoon of finely chopped fresh parsley

1 teaspoon garlic powder

¼ cup of pine nuts

Directions:

Preheat oven to 400 degrees.

Peel the eggplant and cube.

Put cubed eggplant on cookie sheet. Sprinkle with salt and drizzle olive oil to coat.

Toss ingredients in cookie sheet until coated and spread out into an even layer.

Bake eggplant for 15 minutes.

Set aside until cooled down.

Transfer eggplant to a mixing bowl. Mix together with breadcrumbs, eggs, chopped parsley, grated cheese, garlic powder and pine nuts.

Once mixed, roll into meatball shape and place onto parchment lined cookie sheet.

Bake for 15-20 minutes at 350 degrees.

Fried corn

Ingredients:

2 corn on the cob

1 tablespoon of EVOO

Salt

Directions:

Cut corn off of the cob.

Heat EVOO and add corn on medium high heat.

Stir corn occasionally until golden brown, about 5 minutes.

Season with salt to taste.

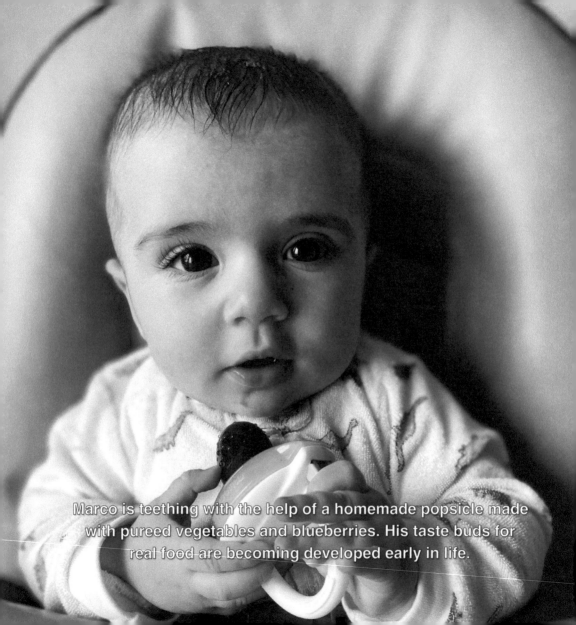

Marco is teething with the help of a homemade popsicle made with pureed vegetables and blueberries. His taste buds for real food are becoming developed early in life.

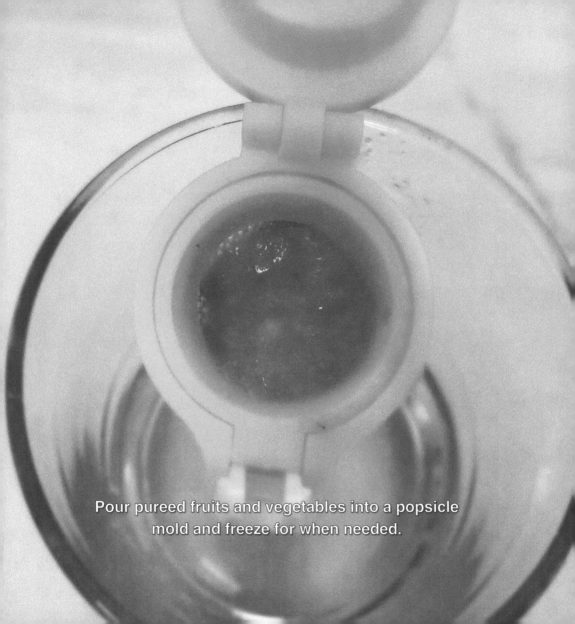
Pour pureed fruits and vegetables into a popsicle mold and freeze for when needed.

Strawberry, Cauliflower and Lemon Popsicle

About 6 florets of fresh cauliflower

¼ cup fresh strawberries

½ t fresh squeezed lemon juice

Place the florets in a small pan and over with just enough baby water. Cook until tender when a fork can easily pierce the cauliflower.

When the cauliflower is tender remove it from the pan but keep the water to add as needed for a smooth consistency.

Place the cauliflower, lemon juice and strawberries in a small blender and blend until smooth.

Pour the mixture in popsicle forms and freeze until needed.

These are great not only as a snack but for teething infants and toddlers.

Note; substitute blueberries or other fruit to make a variety of tastes.

Chapter 5:
Tips and comments for
successful outcomes

A Few pieces of low-cost equipment Is all that's needed

You don't need expensive and fancy utensils to make great infant and toddler food. Just a few additional pieces of equipment in addition to what you probably already have in your kitchen.

Possibly the most useful piece of equipment for preparing infant food is a blender allowing for quick pureeing and storing of fresh healthful baby food. Having additional small bowls for the blender allows for batch preparation of foods which can remain fresh for at least a couple of days in your refrigerator. When finished blending, just place the cap on top of the blender bowl and either store in the refrigerator until needed. Preparing and storing of food a couple of times a week is easy and economical. This type of preparation allows for controlling exactly what goes into the baby's food with no hidden addition of additives or using high heat killing nutrients. A quick online search will turn up no less than 7 different types and brands of small blenders ranging in price from $39.95 to $149.99.

Another very useful gadget is a mold for making your child tasty "popsicles" using fruits and vegetables. See photo on page 78. Frozen popsicles are wonderful as a snack and for teething. Little Marco on page 77 is enjoying a blueberry popsicle in his highchair. He's getting his daily intake of antioxidants from the blueberries while teething and developing his taste for healthful fruit. An online search will most likely turn up a dozen different popsicle molds ranging in price from $4.99 to $36.99.

Preserve or develop a food culture that lasts a lifetime and beyond

Families with backgrounds from healthful food cultures may have an advantage if they are preserving their culture while linking food and family traditions. If, however, ancient food cultures are abandoned for the standard American diet (SAD) the benefits from the culture of origin are lost. Perhaps a re-connection with healthful foods your parents, grandparents or relatives served is all that's needed. Hopefully it's easy enough to re-visit the types of fresh foods that were prepared from the garden a few generations ago. Unfortunately, the SAD diet begins to replace the diet of our ancestors in just one generation. You will not only become reacquainted with familial foods but probably some wonderful traditions connected with food as well when you return to our original culture.

Families without ancient food cultures in their background have an opportunity to build one. For example, engaging young children in gardens, seeing food growing, touching, smelling and having real food experiences with family and friends develops both a food education as well as special lasting childhood memories combining food, culture and family.

The photos in the book of Nico and Lorenzo convey a compelling story of introducing young children to real food while becoming involved with helping to prepare it. Early memories from our past become part of each of us. It's a gift to provide those fond memories about food to our children as well. Allow your children to enjoy the pleasures of eating food that is lovingly prepared and shared with friends and family. Early involvement with helping prepare food introduces them to giving to the family and not just taking from others.

It's never too early to educate on the perils of eating processed, sugary and artificially flavored manufactured food. While small children may enjoy sugary foods from time to time at birthday parties or other events, we can instill knowledge that fresh foods made a home is what will create and maintain their health. It's also not too early to let children know that what's in the pretty colored boxes of food in the grocery store are not the best types of food that will help them grow big and strong.

When considering the increase in childhood obesity and other chronic illnesses in the U.S. and the world, it's easy to conclude there has never been a more pressing time to introduce children to food in its purest form early in life and developing a palate for it. Sadly, based upon serial NHANES (National Health and Nutrition Examination) surveys of nutritional status of adults and children from 1999 to 2016, the estimated overall diet quality of children in the U.S. showed more than half of youths age 2 - 19 had poor-quality diets. We can reverse this trend in our very own kitchens!

Feeding infants and toddlers doesn't have to be complicated and families do not have to become nutritionists to be successful. Even though I am a nutritionist and I love the science of nutrition, I've also observed that too much focus on individual nutrients, or the latest discovery about nutrition can have negative effects. Remember, real food remains simple. There is no need to get fussy or obsessive.

One last thought that cannot be overlooked. Your part as the role model is extremely important. If the adults in a child's life are eating heavily processed and fast foods such as processed meats, sugar, saturated fats and artificially flavored and sweetened foods it's going to be challenging to introduce real food for the child. What I love about how Italians feed their children in Italy, is that children eat what their parents eat, and their parents are eating real food. For this reason, there is no reason for "kids' menus" in Italy. Food for infants and toddlers begins with the type of recipes in this book and it easily transitions to what parents are eating as well.

Reference:

JAMA. 2020 Mar 24;323(12):1161-1174. doi: 10.1001/jama.2020.0878.

Trends in Diet Quality Among Youth in the United States, 1999-2016.

Liu J[1], Rehm CD[2,3], Onopa J[1], Mozaffarian D[1].

About Carol Amendola D'Anca

Carol D'Anca was raised in a small Wisconsin town steeped in the Italian culture where gardening and home cooked meals in the Neapolitan tradition were common. She became aware of the vast differences in dietary choices within the U.S. early in life, igniting a life-long pursuit of the study of nutrition as it relates to disease.

An honors graduate at the University of WI, she earned her Master of Clinical Nutrition Degree at Rosalind Franklin University of Medicine and Science/The Chicago Medical School. After completing her internship, she became a licensed dietician/nutritionist. Currently Mrs. D'Anca is an active practitioner, author and much sought-after speaker.

Her first book, "Real Food for Healthy People" has achieved status as an Amazon bestselling book. This, her most recent book, "Real Food for Infants and Toddlers" provides quick and easy ways of feeding children nutrient dense foods while helping infants and toddlers develop tastes for natural unprocessed foods that last a lifetime.

Carol's presentations and lectures at medical workshops, conferences, academic settings, private and public organizations in the U.S. and internationally, have helped raise awareness and inspire dietary change for thousands of people in the U.S. and abroad.

About Barbara J. Deal, MD

Barbara J. Deal, MD is Professor of Pediatrics and Getz Chair of Cardiology at Northwestern University, Feinberg School of Medicine. Her educational background includes an undergraduate degree from Duke University, medical degree and residency in pediatrics at Northwestern University and fellowships in Pediatric Cardiology at Boston Children's Hospital and Electrophysiology at the University of Illinois. Dr. Deal is the author of over 100 papers, 28 book chapters and the editor of 2 books. Among her clinical interests is the role of nutrition in cardiovascular disease.

About Raffaella Maiorino Florio

Raffaella Maiorino Florio was born, raised and educated in the region of Campagna Italy. A graduate of the Istituto Tecnico Economico in Salerno Italy, she was married while in Italy and emigrated to the U.S. at the age of 26.

Early in life she was exposed to gardening and cooking spending hours in the kitchen with her mother and grandmother. As the oldest of 4 children she watched her mother making her sisters and brother's infant foods fresh from their garden.

Following the birth of her first child, shortly after arriving in the U.S., Raffaella created infant and toddler foods for her child in the same way she watched her mother preparing them – with fresh ingredients which were minimally processed.

She remains a strong advocate of making baby food at home, avoiding commercial over processing which occurs at high temperatures while destroying vitamins and minerals. Raffaella's guiding principle is to know exactly what you are feeding your baby and to know how it was prepared.

Raffaella lives in RI with her husband, two daughters, sons-in-law and 3 grandsons where she continues preparing meals each day for her family.

Author's Note

My practice is solely focused on whole food plant-based nutrition. When dietary choices are carried out correctly the whole food plant-based approach will deliver the necessary protein, fats, and carbohydrates necessary for a strong foundation for health. As part of the book's collaboration, you will notice a few recipes will include small amounts of egg and cheese leaving the addition or removal of the ingredients to your personal discretion. I know you will enjoy this little book of treasured recipes that have been used for generations.

-Carol Amendola D'Anca MS, LDN, CNS Board Certified

For any questions feel free to contact me at: info@foodnotmeds.com.

Additional whole food plant based recipes for adults
can be accessed at: www.foodnotmeds.com

CPSIA information can be obtained
at www.ICGtesting.com
Printed in the USA
BVHW021325130720
583608BV00001B/46